Autism
Theories Dissected
You Are Right!

What we might never have figured out

R.M.Terry

R M Terry

Copyright © 2014 R. M. Terry

Editing by: Cory Scott
Book Cover Design: Diversepixel (Self Pub Book Covers)
Book Cover Design contributor: Dominique Edwards
Publicist: Tavares Cherry
Other: Clarity

ISBN: 1500917974
ISBN-13: 9781500917975

Published by: RM Terry

DEDICATION

I dedicate this research project to my husband by acknowledging his dedication to our son's recovery process.

You were there for every doctor visit, consult, and seminar. You were there through all the diets, supplements, and therapies. Our son may not be recovered yet, but he is definitely much better. He has come a long way from that kid who was 100% nonverbal and couldn't even understand receptive language. I can remember when the only words he understood were "let's eat" and "let's go." His regression from a verbal, chubby, happy, and excited toddler to a nonverbal, thin, unhappy, sickly, and withdrawn toddler was very difficult and overwhelming for us. But we made it through by sticking together and working as a team. Now when he asks for "a few more minutes" of sleep in the morning, we can hardly believe it. Our family's autism journey is not over yet, but I can honestly say that our son is lucky to have you as his father and I am lucky to have you as my husband.

R M Terry

CONTENTS

ACKNOWLEDGMENTS

To the Parents, Family members, Scientists, Doctors, Chiropractors, Medical professionals, Researchers, Teachers, Therapists, Organizations, Friends, and all who have voiced an attempt to help solve this autism puzzle — *You are right!*

Your medical research, blogs, Internet posts, videos, emails, books, articles, and seminars have made me familiar with your theories. Your commitment to this cause is genuine and sincere. I thank you for all you've done because I couldn't have come this far without you.

A special acknowledgement to www.23andme.com.

The health related genetic report that you performed on my son was indispensable to my research. The time and money this $299 dollar genetic screening saved my research is incalculable. At a time when I felt so lost and helpless, you provided information that was not available to me as a parent by any other means. Your genetic screening of over 49 genetic disorders, genetic responses to 25 different drugs, 55 genetic traits, and 106 health risks allowed me to get to know my son in a way that helped me become an informed health advocate. I was deeply saddened to learn that this test was removed from your panel. Know that your vision to empower consumers with their genetic information made a huge impact on my family's life. I hope that one day you'll win your fight and be able to realize your full vision again.

To everyone committed to stopping this devastating disorder,

Let's keep the information flowing until we

Wipe Out Autism

1 THE COMMON CONNECTION

What is autism?

Is it a psychological disorder?

Is it a genetic disorder that affects the brain and body?

Is it the result of a triggered environmental factor?

Is it all of these?

Autism is especially confounding because of its wide spectrum.

Why are some kids affected mildly and others severely?

Why are some kids born with autism, while most others regress into it at 12-16 months of age?

In this report, I aim to analyze *Regressive Autism.* This type of autism can be described simply as an unexplained medical disorder that causes the developmental deviation of neuro typical appearing babies into stereotypical autistic toddlers. These neuro typical appearing babies usually make their developmental milestones and then after 12 months of age start losing them. Unexplainably within a period of weeks to months they start exhibiting symptoms such as poor eye contact, loss of speech, toe walking, poor socialization, repetitive behavior, sleep dysfunction, issues with sensory processing, poor muscle tone and more.

A crucial question looming in our future is,

Who will care for this vast population of children once they become adults and their parents are no longer around or capable of performing as caregivers?

The question of what will happen to my son when my husband and I are gone motivates me to dedicate my life to learning the causes of autism. I want to know why my son is the way he is. Then I want a doctor to suggest a realistic treatment plan. I hope that my research will give doctors and scientists who are working so diligently to solve this autism puzzle a new direction to consider. Success will come if we can merge everyone's contributions into one cohesive theory. "You Are Right" is a fitting title of this book because everyone is right, but in order to see the connection or algorithm we must share our collective knowledge with the understanding that we are not the only ones who are right.

Step number one, identify the problem.

What actually causes regressive autism?

Most of the families have similar stories: We mothers have some sort of autoimmune disorder ranging from Lupus to allergies (diagnosed or undiagnosed). We each had a child born seemingly neurotypical (some premature, but most of normal gestation age). Most of our babies were bottle fed from the start or weaned early from breast milk for various reasons (latching issues, low production of milk, etc.). Then due to standard infant formula intolerance, the formula was switched to soy-based or pre-digested milk-based formula. Within a few months these babies started to experience frequent upper respiratory or ear infections, and were given multiple courses of antibiotics. Somehow these now toddlers were still meeting their developmental milestones including verbal skills: able to say small words such as "mama" and "dada." They appeared alert, engaged, and played appropriately, not yet showing any stereotypical signs of autism.

Months passed; more upper respiratory and ear infections were treated with antibiotics; then food and environmental allergies started appearing. At one year of age, after switching from infant formula to whole cow milk, milk intolerance quickly became apparent: i.e. loose stools, constipation, gastrointestinal distress, or psoriasis, etc. (My son had bloody stools.) Due to so many illnesses most of these kids were behind in their vaccine schedule. Then between 12-16 months they were given the MMR vaccine along with the missed vaccines and within weeks the regression happened: they stopped speaking, exhibited poor muscle tone, and had issues with sensory processing. Their anxiety attacks started, as well as the long list of stereotypical autistic behaviors that continued as part of their daily lives.

This is my family's story and the story of many others. I see our common story as the major part of this autism puzzle. No one except the parent of an autistic child knows what it feels like to have a beautifully vibrant baby turn into a toddler who seems detached from his environment, almost like a *Zombie*. I don't use that term to be insulting, just as a description of the extreme nature of the personality changes that occurred over a few months' time.

I use *Zombie*, also, because of an incident that occurred in Florida between 1998 and 2003: an ecological mystery as to why hundreds of alligators were dead or dying in

Lake Griffin. Even up to one thousand pound alligators were unable to swim, therefore, were drowning in their own habitat. These alligators had neurological symptoms; they appeared to no longer be aware of their environment. In a documentary, National Geographic named these alligators *Zombie Alligators*. After years of research and the loss of hundreds of alligators, the environmental factor that triggered this phenomenon was found. The cause of the alligators' neurological symptoms and deaths was a simple change in their diet. The normal varieties of fish in Lake Griffin were altered by environmental changes caused by run off from muck farms, which caused algae to bloom out of control. These algae blooms lead to the death of most species of fish, except for one, the Gizzard Shad, which thrived in these conditions. The Gizzard Shad was high in thiaminase, an enzyme that breaks down thiamine or vitamin B1. With a diet exclusively eaten of this thiaminase rich fish, the alligators gradually became vitamin B1 deficient and died of a neurological disorder identified as Beriberi. Armed with this knowledge, researchers were able to supplement vitamin B1, improve the water quality and restock the lake with a variety of fish that were naturally high in vitamin B1. With their cleaned environment, healthy populations of alligators—not *Zombies*—now thrive in Lake Griffin.

To clarify, the point of my telling this true story is not to suggest that our autistic kids are suffering from a simple vitamin B1 deficiency. However, this story does illustrate how something natural that normally belongs in an environment can have detrimental effects if its concentration is too high.

This led me to conclude that "You Are Right!" in your summation as to the contributing causes of the regressive autism epidemic.

You are right; everyone is right because your theories have one thing in common: *Surfactants*.

To the epidemiologists, ecologists, environmentalists, microbiologists, scientists, doctors, and parents trying to complete our autism puzzles, here we go...

Ten most probable causes of autism and learning disabilities
(Mount Sinai School of Medicine)

1. Lead
2. Methyl mercury
3. PCB - polychlorinated biphenyl
4. Organophosphate pesticides
5. Organochlorine pesticides
6. Endocrine disrupters
7. Automotive exhaust
8. Polycyclic aromatic hydrocarbons
9. Brominated flame retardants
10. Perflourinated compounds

Source of list: Icahn School of medicine at Mt. Sinai April 25, 2012

Items on this list connected to surfactants

PCB – Production of this chemical was banned in the U.S. in 1979 due to its detrimental effect on the environment. PCB's were put in dielectric and coolant fluids, insecticides, paints, varnish, lacquer, plastics, lubricants, inks, adhesives, caulking compounds and more.

It's now 35 years later and the PCB cleanup process is still going on. One of the ways PCB's are cleaned up is with the use of surfactants.

Pesticides: Surfactants are added to pesticides as adjuvants to help the chemicals absorb better.

Endocrine disrupters: Surfactants are endocrine disrupters.

Automotive exhaust: Surfactants are added to gasoline as detergents, dispersants, corrosion inhibitors, carburetor cleaners and anti-icers.

Polycylic aromatic hydrocarbons: Surfactants are added as adjuvants (examples: vehicle exhaust, asphalt roads, roofing tar, plastics, pesticides and more)

Brominated flame retardants: Surfactants are added as adjuvants.

Perflourinated compounds: surfactants are added as adjuvants (examples from flourosurfactant list: - nonstick cookware, stain resistant carpet, paint, adhesives, foamers, cleaners, polishes, waxes and more.

*adjuvants are items added to substances in order to aide, assist or enhance it.

R M Terry

2 HERBICIDE/ PESTICIDE/POLLUTION/ ENVIRONMENTAL - THEORIES

One of the most common autism theories is that it is caused by environmental factors. However, public awareness of surfactant exposure is poor. Surfactants are commonly used in chemical, manufacturing, pharmaceutical, and food industries. Because it remains under the radar, no one knows the exact health effects of exposure to toxic levels of surfactants.

Surfactants, by definition, are compounds that lower the surface tension between two liquids or a liquid and a solid. These compounds are made up of phospholipids (fats) and proteins. Our lungs make their own surfactants in order to lower the surface tension in our alveoli allowing our lungs to expand so that we can breathe. Surfactants, which include surfactant proteins A, B, C, and D, are very important because they help us with innate host defense or immunity. So surfactants are part of our normal environment. We know that when lungs don't make enough surfactant the immune system suffers, which makes us vulnerable to opportunistic infections and asthma-like symptoms.

Types of surfactants used in chemical, manufacturing, pharmaceutical, and food industries include: Anionic, Cationic, Amphoteric, and Nonionic Surfactants.

Herbicide formulas (for commercial or home use) usually use nonionic <u>surfactants</u> as <u>additives</u> or <u>adjuvants</u>. The more surfactant added to herbicides the better they work; the formulas contain up to 50% surfactants. By definition, surfactants decrease the surface tension between two liquids and a liquid and a solid. The ability to decrease the surface tension on the leaves of a plant allows the chemical to coat the leaves and achieve better penetration. Herbicides then saturate the soil and are swept down into the sewers, rivers, and lakes as runoff when it rains. Environmentalists have complained about the negative health effects of herbicides for many years. Most of us, me included, have turned deaf ears to their warnings by prioritizing lawn beautification over health. That is, of course, until the damage is done to our health and our symptoms lead us to switch to organic products. Synthetic and natural (coconut based) surfactants are listed as being biodegradable, therefore, assumed to be harmless to humans and animals.

But to what extent?

Pesticides – Few people like bugs, which can be scary and a nuisance. Some damage crops, thereby affecting food supplies and causing financial hardships for farmers. So we get rid of bugs by killing them with pesticides. Like in herbicides, synthetic and natural <u>surfactants</u> help pesticides penetrate. Some manufacturers stopped adding surfactants directly to their formulas, but instruct buyers to add them because without surfactants their products won't work well.

Pollution – Air pollution is a known environmental hazard. Government agencies create programs to improve air quality to reduce negative health effects triggered by pollution. So many sources of air pollution exist that I focus on *automotive exhaust*, which is on the Mount Sinai Medical School list as a probable cause of autism. Thirty years ago, having one vehicle in the driveway was enough; the head of the family usually had the vehicle and transported the others wherever they needed to go. Now, four cars in the driveway could be considered the norm for a family with four members of driving age. Another change to our normal habitat is that we live with our cars: we park them in our attached garages, not considering the effects of the chemicals that are off gassing from them directly into our homes.

<u>Surfactants</u> are added to gasoline as detergents, dispersants, corrosion inhibitors, carburetor cleaners, and anti-icers.

Does anyone know the health effects of breathing in surfactants mixed in exhaust fumes?

Environment – <u>Surfactants</u> are used in our living environments: daily we are probably exposed to more than 100 different surfactants in our homes (a conservative estimate). Because they improve the soaping and foaming actions, surfactants are in most cleaning products as well as most hair and bathing products; some contain more than 15 different surfactants.

How bad is your family's exposure to surfactants?

Why not take your own survey?

Read the back label of every product you use during a 24-hour period. Ninety nine percent of these ingredients won't be labeled as surfactants. Instead they will have long chemical unrecognizable names among the names of other ingredients. This list of surfactants is too long (thousands) for me to put in this report. The best approach for being able to recognize a surfactant is to have your Smart Phone or computer handy when you check your labels. Type all unknown names in an internet search engine and cross-reference them with the word "surfactant." For example, if you search for "Ammonium Lauryl Sulfate," a description comes up; read the description to make sure that it is indeed a surfactant.

Here is a <u>partial list</u> of surfactants from the back label of **one** bottle of shampoo: ammonium lauryl sulfate, ammonium laureth sulfate, disodium cocoaamphodipropionate, cocoamide cea, trideceth-7 carboxylic acid, glycol distearate, laureth-10, sodium laureth sulfate, polyquaternium-7, PPG-5-ceteth-10 phosphate, lauramide glucoside, lauryl glucoside, polyquaternium-10, cocoglucoside, glyceryl oleate, disodium EDTA (used as an anionic surfactant), PEG-8 dimethicone, sulfated castor oil (used as an anionic surfactant), lecithin (not a mistake—a surfactant).

Some other surfactants frequently listed in various products and medications are Tween 80, Triton X-100, and Polysorbate 80. But the list seems endless.

Our grandparents used lye-based soaps that were cured over a couple of months in order for the lye to dissipate naturally. Surfactants provide a quicker and cheaper production process. When researching autism, I always ask myself,

What changes have been incorporated in our life style compared to previous generations?

Which products contain surfactants?

1. Toothpaste

2. Mouth wash

3. Hand soap

4. Bath soap – This is one of the biggest offenders because we like bubbles. (I challenge you to find **one** bar of soap in your local supermarket that doesn't contain a surfactant or a multitude of them.)

5. Baby wipes

6. Bubble bath

7. Shampoo – This includes baby shampoos. (Good luck finding one without surfactants!) Sodium lauryl sulfate (SLS) is probably the only surfactant that the general public avoids due to its harsh stripping of fatty acids dries out the hair.

8. Hair conditioner

9. Hair mousse/styling products

10. Lotions/skin creams

11. Dishwashing liquid

12. Washing powder - liquid and powder versions

13. Fabric softener

14. Bathroom cleaners - even organic and all natural—may use a coconut-based surfactant, but still adds to daily surfactant exposure

15. Household cleaners - even organic and all natural—may use a coconut-based surfactant, but still adding to daily surfactant exposure

16. Bug spray, gardening supplies, degreasers, etc. – (Check chemical cabinets - most likely every product contain surfactants or a combination of surfactants.)

17. Spray cans, jugs, etc. - (Check the garage and basement - these products off gas or evaporate; therefore, even if the containers are closed, their gasses may penetrate the container walls and pollute your living environment.)

18. Spermicides – (This one surprised me.) Common spermicides inserted vaginally and added to condoms are indeed surfactants. They disrupt the lipid layer on the tail of the sperm decreasing their motility. Surfactants also alter the fructolytic activity of sperm, which prevents them from utilizing fructose, which is required for survival.

Surfactants are most likely in every brand of these products in the home. The list of daily surfactant exposure goes on and on.

What happens when the human body is exposed to too much surfactant, especially the synthetic surfactants present in the products mentioned above?

Does the body slow down the production of its own natural surfactant and instead try to metabolize available synthetic surfactants?

Is there such thing as surfactant toxicity?

Can exposure to too much surfactant cause surfactant resistance?

Would this disorder work like what is seen in insulin resistance?

Could surfactant resistance lead to a deficiency creating respiratory symptoms and immune system shut down?

Could too much surfactant overstimulate the immune system causing autoimmune disorders?

Could synthetic surfactant toxicity lower the surface tension of the lungs too much causing poor muscle tone (floppy lungs) leading to poor gas exchange? (Did hyperbaric oxygen therapy help many of our kids by increasing their lungs surface tension?)

Could this poor gas exchange then lead to issues with the heart, poor cerebral perfusion and metabolic issues?

Is it also possible for surfactant toxicity to cause an immune system to create antiphospholipid antibodies since surfactants are made of phospholipids?

What would that syndrome look like? How would that affect the ability of our body to metabolize phosphatidylcholine and fatty acids?

How would surfactants affect the blood brain barrier (BBB)?

Currently we have more questions than answers. Right?

Therefore, to you who theorize that herbicides, insecticides, air pollution—multiple environmental factors—are contributing causes of autism, I say, "You Are Right!"

R M Terry

3 NONSTICK COOKWARE/CARPET/BUILDING MATERIALS - THEORIES

For years, nonstick cookware, carpet, chemical cleaners, and anything that has to do with remodeling a house has been labeled taboo in regards to exposing it to a child with autism. Six years ago, I took my son to a world famous Autism Treatment Center in Illinois. I was told to remove the above items from my home as part of his treatment plan. I, of course, questioned why? The doctor said that he didn't know the exact reason, but it was strongly suspected that these items might be contributing factors to autism. Two years before our son was born, my husband and I purchased a newly constructed house with a two-car attached garage, so I removed what I could while, of course, staying in our home.

I have chemical allergies, which were mild until after the birth of my son. Then my chemical allergies to perfumes, pesticides, insecticides, cleaning products, etc. became so bad that I had to avoid certain aisles in grocery and hardware stores. With diet and lifestyle changes, I have improved, but I'll never forget a particularly bad chemical reaction while cleaning my glass dining table. I had already removed cleaning products with harsh chemical from my home and replaced them with organic products. I began to clean the table as usual. As I sprayed organic glass cleaner on it, I had an immediate negative reaction: I felt overwhelmed with noxious chemicals and had to get fresh air immediately. When I was able to return, I turned the bottle around to read what was in it! All the ingredients seemed normal enough, except one—"coconut-derived surfactants." I didn't know what a surfactant was then, but I never forgot the word *surfactant*. Last year while researching herbicides and pesticides I saw *surfactants* again. Then while researching bacteria I saw bio*surfactants*. I began to cross reference everything I had ever been told that may be a contributing factor to autism and noticed that *surfactant* kept coming up. This is how we arrived here at nonstick cookware, carpet, and building materials.

Fluoro<u>surfactant</u> list – (Perflourinated Compounds)

1. Nonstick cookware (PTFE) - polytetrafluoroethylene

2. Carpet stain repellent - formula changed to perfluorobutanesulfnic acid (PFBS) in 2003 after EPA pressure to stop using perfluorooctante sulfonate (PFOS) because of toxicity

3. Paint

4. Adhesives

19

5. Caulking material

6. Waxes

7. Polishes

8. Cleaners

9. Foamers - foam insulation replaced fiber glass insulation in remodeled and new construction homes

10. Vehicle exhaust fuel

Much, much more

Therefore, to those of you who theorize that nonstick cookware, carpet, and building materials are contributing factors to the cause of autism, I say, "You Are Right!"

4 GUT/BACTERIA/ANTIBIOTIC – THEORIES

I love teachers; they taught me that there is no such thing as a stupid question. Most of my questions regarding my son's health issues are received with a blank look or a *What-Are-You-Talking-About?* look. I don't take offence because there are no stupid questions, just questions that can't be answered right now.

Gut dysbiosis is the term used to describe the common GI issues autistic children face. That foul smelling stool is a giveaway that the bacterial bio dome is altered. From special diets to probiotics, we've tried everything to help their little guts. The Gut/Brain connection is well known; it suggests that symbiosis of the gut negates the presence of waste products or toxins that are causing neurological symptoms.

Biosurfactants are bacteria, yeasts, and fungi that make surfactants (it's not just our lungs that make surfactants). An infection with the wrong type of bacteria, yeast, or fungi can turn the body into a surfactant-making factory. One example of a bacterium that produces surfactant rhamnolipids is *Pseudomonas aeruginosa*, and an example of a fungus that produces large amounts of biosurfactant sophorolipids is *Candidas bombicola*. Another member of the Candidas family, *Candidas albicans*, causes a fungal infection well known in the autism community. One common treatment used to kill Candidas is an antifungal macrolide, Nystatin. (We'll talk about the importance of macrolides in chapter 5.)

Here are questions for doctors and scientists:

How would an infection affect the body's overall surfactant production?

Since these bacteria and fungi are producing copious amounts of rhamnolipids and sophorolipids, how would this affect lipid and fatty acid metabolism?

Antibiotics – The double edged sword. These not only kill the bad bacteria, but also keep the good ones from multiplying. When good bacteria are prevented from multiplying we start seeing Candidas fungal infection overgrowth. We can't get away from bacteria, no matter how much we try with our surfactant-filled antibacterial hand soap and our prescription pads. Yes, some may harm us, but most protect us. Dependence on antibiotics has actually led to the antibiotic resistant strains of bacteria that are causing concern to the medical community at large.

Sulfonamide based antibiotics are antibiotics that contain a sulfonamide group in them. They are commonly used to treat babies with bacterial infections as well as babies and kids with ear infections. Two important side effects of this type of antibiotic are that it not only binds to albumin but also disrupts the production of dihydrofolic acid (a type of folic acid).

If folic acid is so important to our children's proper brain development, how would giving sulfonamide based antibiotics affect their brain development?

I'll talk about the significance of antibiotics binding to albumin and autism in chapter 5.

My son received enough antibiotics from age 3 months to 2 years to last him a lifetime. I now am super conservative about taking antibiotics or giving them to my son. (When we know better, we do better.) Now the big talk is about biofilm: how the nastiest, meanest bacteria are creating protective biofilm around themselves to become antibiotic resistant. It is theorized that these biofilm-protected strains are infecting our autistic children.

What if these nasty biofilm-protected bacteria proposed to infect autistic children are the ones producing biosurfactants?

Therefore, to you who theorize that bacteria, fungi, yeast, and antibiotics are contributing factors to the cause of Autism, I say, "You Are Right!"

5 GENETICS/ADRENALS/LUNGS/STEROIDS/ FOOD (SOY, CASEIN, WHEAT)/ALBUMIN/BILIRUBIN/TRYPSIN/ ALPHA 1 ANTI TRYPSIN - THEORIES

Nature vs. Nurture was the argument of the Refrigerator Mom autism theorists of the past. Now, Genetic vs. Environmental factors lead the autism debate. The fact that genetics might play some role in autism is rarely disputed. One just has to wonder why some kids are not affected by autism when all have potentially been exposed to the same environmental factors. Genetics seems the most realistic answer. It has been hypothesized that children who are not affected must have some sort of genetic protection against the offending factors while others seem to have a genetic susceptibility to these unknown factors.

Lungs – In the years 2009 and 2011, St. Joseph's Hospital in Phoenix, Arizona, conducted a study examining the pictures of 459 bronchoscopies done on children. Doctors noticed that 49 of the children had unusual airways: their lower airways branched into doublets, which is not normal. When checking the diagnoses of these children it was noticed that <u>all</u> 49 (100 percent) were diagnosed with autism. This area of the lungs is where our lungs produce <u>surfactants</u>. At present it is not known if this anatomical abnormality is a form of genetic defect.

What would happen if the structure of the lungs were altered?

Is this caused by an undiscovered genetic defect of the lungs or caused by environmental factors?

Lungs – The Scotson technique is a unique physical therapy that uses hand pressure on specific areas of the chest and back to improve oxygenation of the lungs. The theory is that the abnormal development of the lungs and altered breathing patterns contribute to many symptoms of autism. It hypothesizes that altered breathing patterns lead to lowered aerobic metabolism and the buildup of toxic waste products. It also hypothesizes that this is why these children have anxious behaviors, GI issues, immune system problems, poor muscle tone, and lack of speech.

Steroids – Steroids cause the body to make surfactants. Steroids are usually prescribed for autoimmune disorders.

Has anyone researched the amount of steroids mothers have taken prior to the births of their autistic children?

Premature birth is a common risk factor for autism. Steroids are commonly given to pregnant mothers who are at high risk of having premature infants to mature their lungs before birth. They can also be given after birth to help with breathing issues related to poor lung development. Steroids help our children overcome respiratory problems by producing lung surfactant.

But what happens if the body has an increased response to these drugs due to genetics?

"Acute side effects of surfactant treatment" by R. Hentschel and G. Jorch from University Children's Hospital in Freiburg, Germany, should be noted because of the increasing evidence from studies implicating that surfactant administration has a crucial impact on cerebral perfusion. There is no doubt that exogenous surfactant therapy and steroids that help produce surfactants save the lives of premature babies. My son was born at 34 weeks; he received two doses of steroids while in utero in order to help his lung development. But he also has poor cerebral perfusion.

Since long-term side effects aren't clearly known, perhaps should there be some kind of follow up?

Blood Brain Barrier (BBB) – Surfactants can help substances cross the blood brain barrier. Because of this ability, surfactants are used as drug delivery methods in the form of nanoparticles and niosomes.

What toxic chemical substances are now able to cross the blood brain barrier because of increased surfactant exposure?

Are surfactants also allowing waste products like bilirubin easier access to the brain?

Could surfactants therefore be contributing to neurological symptoms in our children by promoting bilirubin encephalopathy?

Adrenals – During the birthing process, the baby's adrenal gland releases the stress hormone cortisol, a steroid that acts as lungs' natural signal to start producing lung surfactants so that the baby can take its first breath. A characteristic common to most children with autism is that they are quite stressed. Anxiety attacks, meltdowns, and obsessive-compulsive behaviors must affect their adrenal glands.

So, what does this mean for their body's natural surfactant production?

Is it up regulated?

What about adrenal fatigue?

Do their adrenals ever just give up and stop sending out the necessary amount of cortisol needed?

What happens to their natural surfactant production then?

Genetics – This is a major factor, and we are starting to get clarity about how genetics may influence autism. It is probably a major reason why some children are affected with autism and others are not. Currently, a clinical trial is testing the theory that a trypsin deficiency could be a contributing cause of some cases of autism. Another genetic disorder, Alpha 1 Antitrypsin deficiency is seen in cystic fibrosis (a lung disorder) cases and has been associated with regressive autism.

The pancreas makes trypsin to break down dietary proteins; the liver makes alpha 1 antitrypsin to protect organs and tissues from being accidentally digested. Alpha 1 antitrypsin deficiency usually manifests as a lung or liver disease, but may also be asymptomatic.

I theorize that mirror image genetic disorders contribute to these autism symptoms. As mirror images, they are complete opposites. Without separating the symptoms of these completely opposite disorders into two groups, findings and treatments would never be totally successful. Trypsin deficiency and alpha 1 antitrypsin deficiency fit that puzzle exactly. Trypsin deficiency would cause hypoalbuminemia due to protein wasting which could then lead to hyperbilirubinemia. While liver disease as seen in alpha 1 antitrypsin deficiency would lead directly to hyperbilirubinemia. This means that treatments that help one condition would be completely intolerable or even harmful to the other.

But what if in some cases trypsin or alpha 1 antitrypsin deficiency's didn't only occur because of a gene deletion or even a gene defect? What if these deficiencies could also be caused by a down regulation of these genes or even a blockage of their gene receptors by surfactants? What if these genes were just turned off?

Infant Formula - One of my strongest clues that connect trypsin and alpha 1 antitrypsin deficiency to autism is infant formula. Babies that have a difficult time digesting standard infant formula are put on a trial of various specialty formulas.

25

There is no science to choosing the formula; the pediatrician recommends the one that is started first. If it doesn't work then a different one is tried. The two types of specialty formulas are soy-based and pre-digested (casein hydrolysate). This is important because soy protein is very high in alpha 1 antitrypsin; pre-digested milk based formula has trypsin added to break down the casein proteins.

That said, what if these children were born with alpha 1 antitrypsin deficiency and others were born with trypsin deficiency? (These genes turned off or receptors blocked by surfactant toxicity)

What if the infant formula supplemented these deficiencies, preventing their becoming symptomatic until, at the standard one-year of age when their formula was replaced with milk? Could removing this support have caused their immune systems to crash, preventing them from being able to handle normal environmental insults?

Food Supply – Many changes have occurred in our food supplies in the past 30 years. With the addition of processed foods comes a very, very long list of preservatives. Most processed foods also contain milk, casein (milk protein), soy, and wheat. The amount of soy and milk protein introduced into our food supply and added to our supplements is mind boggling. Only a person who is sensitive to soy or milk and struggling to find food products without these added ingredients realize how prevalent this is.

Gluten and casein-free diets are often recommended for children with autism. Some theories claim that peptides or proteins cross the blood brain barrier leading to some neurological symptoms of autism. But not all children are positive for gluten or casein sensitivities. So I have to wonder if another protein could cause this problem. I like to look at algorithms or connections: When I think of gluten and casein, I think of wheat and milk. When I think of wheat and milk, I think of their proteins that so many are sensitive to. When I look for a connection between wheat and milk proteins, I think of albumin. When I think of albumin, I think of my son's egg white allergy and my soy sensitivity.

So, that leads me to ask,

Why isn't anyone talking about the albumin and autism connection?

Protein sensitivities common in children with autism

Wheat (wheat proteins – <u>albumin</u>, globulin, gliadin and gluten)

Milk (milk proteins – alpha lact<u>albumin</u>, beta-lactoglobulin, immunoglobulins,
serum <u>albumin</u> and casein)
Soy (soy protein – <u>albumin</u>)
Egg allergy (egg white proteins – albumen/made up of <u>albumin</u> proteins)

So, albumin is the common factor in the most common protein sensitivities in children with autism.

This then leads to questions regarding the surfactant/albumin ratio and the immune system:

If a child has an issue with both surfactants and albumin due to allergies, genetic defects or environmental influences, how would that affect the surfactant/albumin ratio necessary for proper lung development?

How would that affect the immune system?

Could an albumin allergy lead to autoimmune hemolytic anemia?

*How would an albumin allergy affect how bilirubin is removed from the body since bilirubin needs available albumin to bind to for removal?

Bilirubin encephalopathy is a neurological disorder that **looks exactly like autism**. It is caused by bilirubin a blood waste product crossing the blood brain barrier and damaging the brain. Symptoms include auditory processing dysfunction, high pitched crying/vocalizations, speech deficit, oculomotor impairments (nystagmus, strabismus, impaired upward or downward gaze or corticol visual impairment), abnormal motor control, abnormal muscle tone (decreased or increased) and in some cases a dysplasia of the enamel of deciduous teeth (baby teeth) is seen.

Kernicterus is a severe type of bilirubin encephalopathy caused by bilirubin toxicity to the brain.

Could some of our kids actually have a subtle form of Kernicterus like seen in subtle bilirubin encephalopathy (SBE)?

Or even a chronic form of bilirubin encephalopathy like seen in chronic bilirubin encephalopathy?

Risk factors to Kernicterus: G6PDD, Gilbert's syndrome, Rh incompatibility, premature birth, Crigler-Najjar syndrome type I, polycythemia and sulfonamides which includes certain antibiotics (displaces bilirubin from albumin). I also add trypsin deficiency due to its hypoalbuminemia effect and alpha 1 anti trypsin deficiency due to its hyperbilirubinemia effect.

To help you understand the importance of adding bilirubin to your autism puzzle I would like to share with you a letter I wrote to www.G6PDD.org on November 2, 2011 which was posted on their website regarding this subject:

Hello,

I really want to thank you for the important work that you do as well as listening to my story.

Since you said your wife is interested in looking into the relationship between Autism and G6PDD I thought I should send you both my full theory.

I think this Autism Epidemic is caused by an increased incidence of Kernicterus caused by pharmaceutical drug induced hemolytic anemia. Therefore Autism is Kernicterus. This means that people with G6PDD, Gilbert's syndrome and Crigler-Najjar Syndrome type I and II are at risk for being diagnosed with Autism.

I believe that the method of medical treatment that has changed over the last 40 years has created this epidemic. IE, Antibiotic abuse, Vitamin K at birth, Increase in immunizations.

What we know is that in G6PDD the contraindicated drugs bind to Albumin receptors. When hemolytic crisis occurs the Bilirubin level goes up causing Jaundice. Because the Albumin receptors are already bound with the drug, the bilirubin that is supposed to bind with the Albumin receptors has nothing to bind to. This leads to too much FREE bilirubin circulating in the blood. This crosses the blood brain barrier and creates the symptoms of Autism which are exactly like Kernicterus and thereby causing "Autism". I think that these children are not exhibiting the normal clues of Jaundice and are therefore never caught in time, ie yellow skin and eyes. Medical literature states that you should not diagnose Jaundice by visual methods alone, because it does not always present that way.

Medical literature also states that when you already have a hemolytic disease that it does not take extremely high bilirubin levels to cause Kernicterus. Because it is the amount of FREE bilirubin that counts. It is also interesting to note that there is no standard test to check FREE bilirubin levels. This means that most doctors are just looking at standard levels. Here is an abstract explaining the importance. http://fn.bmj.com/content/93/5/F384.abstract

I believe the reason why there is such a spectrum in Autism is because the damage would depend on how much FREE bilirubin was available for each child, how quickly their body could manage the problem, how many immunizations they were given at once and how weak their body was before the immunization. Some children like my son were given multiple courses of antibiotics on your contraindicated list weeks before the immunization due to recurrent ear infections. (This is a common story). Therefore their bodies could have already been experiencing hemolysis and the immunization just took them over the edge. (This is the common story).

All of us parents are saying the same thing about what caused our child's autism. (Immunizations), but is it also Antibiotics that play a part for this sensitive population?

Of course all children that have G6PD, Gilbert's syndrome, Crigler-Najjar Syndrome type I and II do not get Kernicterus. But maybe these lucky children also have some type of Genetic protection that helps them clear their bilirubin faster.

I theorize that there is a small window of opportunity to check and save these children. First you have to actually SCREEN for G6PDD at birth. (Before giving the standard protocol of Vitamin K within 1 hour of life). Then if positive, use all natural means to treat ear infections instead of antibiotics. Also if the parents choose to immunize, check bilirubin levels multiple times starting at 24 hours after immunization to assess hemolysis. Most importantly doctors need to do the calculations to check FREE bilirubin level. Here is calculator on how to calculate FREE bilirubin http://criglernajjar.altervista.org/treb.htm

Remember bilirubin levels should be normal if no active hemolysis is happening for G6PDD, so you would only be able to check during an actual hemolytic crisis.

Could my theory be the connection that explains why children born in winter months are more likely to get Autism?

http://www.ucdmc.ucdavis.edu/publish/news/cvc/5250

My Kernicterus/ bilirubin theory would mean that mother nature tries to take care of this problem by reducing bilirubin levels naturally with sunlight. (This is why every hospital uses bililights in the NICU to reduce bilirubin levels).

Therefore in winter months there is less sunlight; therefore more children wouldn't get this protection.

Please feel free to pass this theory on to your Forum.

Thanks,

RM Terry

In 2011 I didn't have my surfactant piece to this puzzle therefore surfactants weren't mentioned in the above letter. But by adding it in, autism now appears to be a disorder caused by a weakened blood brain barrier (caused by surfactants) and neurological problems caused by bilirubin encephalopathy. Bilirubin encephalopathy may be the result of undiagnosed blood disorders causing hemolysis, undiagnosed liver disorders causing hyperbilirubinemia, undiagnosed disorders causing hypoalbuminemia or side effects of any drug that blocks albumin receptors which leads to hyperbilirubinemia.

Bilirubin's dependence on available albumin for disposal is the critical piece to this puzzle. As stated in the above letter certain drugs bind to albumin receptors preventing albumin from being available to bind to bilirubin when needed for disposal. These drugs reduce the amount of free or available albumin needed to remove bilirubin which increases the chance for it to cross the blood brain barrier causing negative neurological effects **ranging from acute, chronic or subtle bilirubin encephalopathy**. I believe this range of bilirubin encephalopathy is actually the range of our autism spectrum disorder, with most of our kids falling into the chronic or subtle bilirubin encephalopathy categories. I think the problem lies in the word **kernicterus** which is seen in acute bilirubin encephalopathy. I believe everyone is looking for the severest cases and therefore missing the subtle cases of this disorder.

This may be why drug side effects causing hyperbilrubinemia are missed if the obvious sign of jaundice isn't present.

Blocking of albumin receptors is a common side effect of most drugs. However each drug has different levels of binding affinity from low to high. Sulfonamide based antibiotics which are commonly used to treat ear infections have a high affinity to bind albumin.

Gilberts and G6Pdd are what doctors call comorbid diseases. This just means that it is common to see both of these diseases in the same person. So imagine that you have a child with a bleeding disorder like G6Pdd which causes hemolysis of his red blood cells which leads to an increased amount of bilirubin in the blood. Then this same child has Gilbert's syndrome a liver disorder that diminishes the liver's ability to remove bilirubin from the body. Now imagine what would happen if this child was given sulfonamide based antibiotics and exposed to too much surfactant which opens the blood brain barrier. This would appear to be the perfect setup or storm for bilirubin encephalopathy.

G6Pdd is more prevalent than most people and doctors are aware of. It is estimated that this disorder affects 10% of African Americans and over 400 million people worldwide.

Gilbert's syndrome is also more prevalent than most people and doctors are aware of. It affects up to 7% of Americans, up to 10% of the general population, and up to 25% of the African population.

These are high numbers; shouldn't all babies be standardly tested for these disorders at birth so that preventative measure can be taken to prevent the detrimental effects of hyperbilirubinemia on the developing brain?

Between 2008 and 2014 autism rates have risen nationwide from 1 in 88 to 1 in 68 children being affected (a 30% increase). In 2014 the states with the highest prevalence of autism are New Jersey with a rate of 1 in 45 children (boys 1 in 28) and Utah with 1 in 46 children. Alabama has the lowest incidence with a rate of 1 in 175 children affected with autism. As variable as these rates are state to state, there are two communities whose variance is even more puzzling. These communities are the Amish and Somali (African) communities. In the Amish community autism is almost nonexistent (estimated rate of 1 in 271). In the Somali community of Minneapolis Minnesota autism rates are 1 in 32 children. Even though Somalis make up a minority of the Minneapolis population, (approx. 6% of children in school district) they make up the highest number of total kids with autism in these school districts.

Why is this Somali community affected so hard?
Why are New Jersey and Utah affected so hard? Why is the Amish community protected?
Why is Alabama protected?

Based on the research presented in the book I aim to answer these questions with these proposed Autism formulas:

Autism Formula #1

Undiagnosed hemolytic blood disorders and/or undiagnosed hyper bilirubin causing disorders + level of surfactant exposure and/or genetic defect of surfactant proteins ABC or D.
= opened blood brain barrier and bilirubin neurotoxicity (Autism)

Autism Formula #2

Level of surfactant exposure and/ or genetic defect of surfactant proteins ABC or D. + sulfonamide based antibiotics (or any drug that blocks albumin receptors) or disorder that causes hypoalbuminemia + undiagnosed bleeding disorder
= opened blood brain barrier and bilirubin neurotoxicity (Autism)

List of possible undiagnosed bleeding disorders:

Hemophilia – affects mostly males (listed as rare and appears to affect all races equally)

G6Pdd – affects mostly males (most common gene defect in world which affects all races but most common in African, Asian and Mediterranean populations)

Autoimmune hemolytic anemia – listed as rare, but anyone who has an autoimmune disorder knows how difficult it is to get diagnosed with one. Most people go from doctor to doctor without success, trying to figure out what is causing their odd symptoms.

Alpha thalassemia – affects mostly males (listed as rare)

Von Willebrand disease – affects males and females (most common bleeding disorder in America)

List of possible undiagnosed liver disorders causing hyper bilirubinemia:

Gilbert's syndrome – affects men and women, but mostly men with up to a 7:1 ratio (very common disorder with incidence up to 7% of U.S. population and up to 25% of African population)

Crigler Najjar syndrome Type I and II- affects males and females (listed as extremely rare)

Dubin Johnson syndrome – is a rare disorder that affects people of all ethnic backgrounds, but is more prevalent in people with Iranian or Moroccan Jewish heritages.

Rotor syndrome – is consider a rare disorder, however prevalence is unknown.

Biliary obstruction – can be caused by infection or weakened immune system.

Liver damage – possibilities range from genetics to drugs like antibiotics and certain fever reducing drugs that damage the liver.

List of other possible undiagnosed disorders that can lead to hyperbilirubinemia

Alpha 1 anti –trypsin deficiency – listed as one of the most common inherited disorders among white people. This disorder is often misdiagnosed as asthma.

Trypsin deficiency – Prevalence not listed

It is assumed that a person with one of the above disorders would be diagnosed; however most of these disorders have symptoms that range from severe to mild or even asymptomatic. Also when a person has another diagnosed disorder that takes precedence like autism, it may be difficult to distinguish the symptoms of another disorder with milder presentation.

Autism cluster:

Autism rates in *Minneapolis* Minnesota in 2009 showed that 1 in 48 children had autism (not updated for 2014 rates). This average was created from statistics of Somali (sub Saharan African) immigrants having a rate of 1 in 32, whites 1 in 36, African American (non Somali) 1 in 62 and Hispanic 1 in 80.

Notice the change in demographic pattern in Minneapolis. Previously in the United States whites have always been known to have the highest incidence of autism, but now in Minneapolis this has changed.

What could have happened to cause such high rates of autism in the Somali community? This high incidence of autism does not appear to be occurring in their homeland. Could genetics, increased surfactant exposure, increased antibiotic usage, and increased immunization requirements be causative factors?

Proposed cause of increased Somoli risk:

Gilbert's syndrome and/or G6Pdd + Environmental surfactant exposure
= weakened blood brain barrier and bilirubin neurotoxicity (Autism)

or

Gilbert's syndrome and/or G6Pdd + Drug side effects/binding albumin receptors
(antibiotics etc.) + Environmental surfactant exposure
= weakened blood brain barrier and bilirubin neurotoxicity (Autism)

Since Gilbert's syndrome is seen in up to 25% of the Somali population and G6Pdd is seen in over 30% of the sub Saharan African population these disorders would be highly suspect.

Proposed cause of decreased Amish risk:

Diagnosed hyperbilirubin causing genetic disorder - Common environmental
surfactant exposure = Autism protection

Example:

Crigler-Najjar Syndrome (diagnosed) - Common environmental surfactant exposure
= Autism protection

Although extremely rare, Crigler-Najjar syndrome (causing hyperbilirubinemia) is more common in Amish communities and diagnosed and treated early to prevent kernicterus. The Amish also have less environmental surfactant exposure than the rest of the nation because they make their own soaps and detergents out of lye. They are also less likely to purchase the common day products filled with surfactants (refer back to product list on page 15). Surfactant filled air pollution exposure is also reduced because the Amish don't drive cars. This also means they don't live with their cars like the rest of us with our attached garages.

Proposed cause of increased New Jersey risk:

Undiagnosed hemolytic blood disorders and/or undiagnosed hyper bilirubin causing liver disorders + <u>high</u> level of surfactant exposure and/or genetic defect of surfactant protein ABC or D
= opened blood brain barrier and bilirubin neurotoxicity (Autism)
or

Undiagnosed hemolytic blood disorders and/or undiagnosed hyper bilirubin causing liver disorders + Drug side effects/binding albumin receptors (antibiotics etc.) +<u>high</u> level of surfactant exposure and/ or genetic defect of surfactant protein ABC or D
= opened blood brain barrier and bilirubin neurotoxicity (Autism)

In New Jersey the environmental surfactant component stands out. New Jersey has the highest number of surfactant, detergent and chemical manufactures in the United States. Waste disposal from these manufactures as well as products directly purchased to be used in the home would increase surfactant exposure to these residents.

Proposed increased Utah risk:

<u>Undiagnosed hyper bilirubin causing liver disorders</u> and/or undiagnosed hemolytic blood disorder + high level of surfactant exposure and/or genetic defect of surfactant proteins ABC or D
= opened blood brain barrier and bilirubin neurotoxicity (Autism)

or

<u>Undiagnosed hypoalbuminemia causing disorder</u> and/or undiagnosed hemolytic blood disorder + Drug side effects/binding albumin receptors (antibiotics etc.) +high level of surfactant exposure and/ or genetic defect of surfactant proteins ABC or D
= opened blood brain barrier and bilirubin neurotoxicity (Autism)

Utah has its fair share of surfactant, detergent and chemical manufacturers, but they don't have nearly as many of these factories as seen in New Jersey. Nevertheless their rates are the second highest diagnosed autism cases in the United States. Could genetics play a bigger role in this state's high numbers?

In the 1980's there was a study done of 1240 adults in Utah assessing the risk of coronary artery disease (CAD) in relation to bilirubin levels. It was determined that the lower the bilirubin levels the higher the risk of CAD. It was also determined that the higher the bilirubin levels the lower risk of CAD and the lower the cholesterol level because bilirubin seems to increase cholesterol clearance.

This study was meant to show evidence of a major gene (non Gilbert's) that could be causing the higher bilirubin levels in 12% of the study group. Even though these bilirubin levels were not considered excessively high like seen in Gilbert's syndrome, they did show that 12% of the study group has an abnormal increase in bilirubin.

Utah's demographics of a 91% white population would put them at higher incidence of genetic disorders that affect mainly whites.

Since alpha 1 anti trypsin deficiency affects mostly whites, could it also play a role in this population's increase in bilirubin levels?

More about albumin:

Adding albumin to the autism theory creates an entirely new pathway through the immune system involving globular proteins and globulins.

Albumin is a globular protein and a blood transport protein. Not so coincidentally, other members of the albumin blood transport protein family include **GcMAF**/vitamin D binding protein, **alpha-fetoprotein**, and **afamin**/vitamin E binding protein.

Could vitamins D/E binding proteins be another part of my mirror image autism theory?

GcMAF seems to help one subset of kids with autism improve or even recover, but not another. Could afamin be the blood transport protein the other subset of children need? Since GcMAF is in the albumin family of blood transport proteins. Could it be also unblocking albumin receptors? Could afamin also reset the immune system and unblock a different set of albumin receptors? What if another subset of kids needs both GcMAF and afamin to reset their immune systems and unblock their receptors?

Storage Albumin - (hemp seed/cannabis). I included this because I saw a taping of the 2014 Autism One Conference. The endocannabinoid system was mentioned in the same speech as GcMAF. Cannobidiol is a cannabinoid seen in cannabis, it has been known to alleviate self-injurious and violent behaviors in some children with autism.

Could albumin be the connection as to why GcMAF and cannabis help some chldren with autism?

Globulins

- Alpha 1 globulins: **Alpha 1 antitrypsin (Here it is again!)**, Alpha 1 antichymotrypsin, Orsomucoid, Serum amyloid A, Alpha 1 lipoprotein.

- Alpha 2 globulins: Haptoglobin, Alpha-2u globuli, Alpha macroglobulin, ceruloplasmin, Thyroxine binding globulin, Alpha 2 antiplasmin, Protein C, Alpha 2 Lipoprotein, Angiotensinogen
- Beta globulins: beta 2 microglobulin, plasminogen, angiostatins, properdin, sex hormone binding globulin, transferrin

- Gamma globulins: Immunoglobulins Igs (Hypergammaglobulinemia and Hypogammaglobuminemia)

Seeing the above list of globulins takes me back through so many of your autism theories.

Another connection to surfactants and Albumin – Lecithins are surfactants. Egg lecithins, soy lecithins, and sunflower lecithins are most frequently used in wheat products as a dough softener. Therefore, wheat products which are naturally high in albumin protein routinely have surfactant additives.

Is this why so many autistic kids need to be on wheat free diets? Was it actually the albumin and surfactants, not gluten causing their sensitivity symptoms?

What has changed over previous generations? I read that genetically modified wheat has more gluten protein than in previous generations; does it also have more albumin protein in it?

GcMAF/MRT - Some great autism treatments are on the horizon. One treatment now available (not covered by insurance at the time of this writing) is showing great results. It combines Gc protein derived macrophage activating factor (GcMAF or Vitamin D binding protein) with magnetic resonance therapy (MRT). This combination therapy appears to reset the immune system and normalize brain waves, thereby reducing autism symptoms. Early results of this 28 patient double blind study show that 80% of the children have at least 30% improvement in autism symptoms, while 40% are reclassified as neurotypical, based on the Childhood Autism Rating Scale (CARS) score after only 10 weeks of treatment. These are very impressive and exciting results. However, 20% of the children fall into the non-responder group.

My son did a trial of GcMAF last year (not a double-blind study) but was a non-responder. We didn't try MRT because of the cost, but I wonder if he would have been in that unlucky 20% non-responder group and if he is one of the kids that may benefit from my afamin/vitamin E binding protein theory.

Since deep brain stimulation seems to be an effective treatment for some children with Kernicterus, would MRT be considered a less invasive substitute for Kernicterus?

Autophagy – Recently, my brother called me because he saw a report on the news that a new autism treatment is on the horizon. The treatment is testing the well-known Brain Autophagy Autism theory: that people with autism are missing genes that help the body clean up or prune back extra cells. In the case of autism, they are talking about brain synapses which handle communication signals within itself. Having too many or too few synaptic connections causes difficulty in the brain's transmission of information. The drug being investigated as a possible future treatment is a non-antibiotic macrolide named rapamycin. It is already being used to treat cystic fibrosis, which is thought to be an autophagy-mediated disorder that is seen in alpha 1 antitrypsin deficient patients.

But with my mirror image theory, I also believe there may be a subset of kids who have too much autophagy and fall into the too few synaptic connections category.

*GcMAF (Macrophage activation factor) also activates autophagy.

List of Macrolides

Non antibiotic macrolides – sirolimus (rapamycin), tacrolimus and pimecrolimus

Antifungal macrolides – nystatin (common autism treatment), amphotericin B and polyene antimycotics.

Antibiotic macrolides – erythromycin, clarithromycin, azithromycin (only one that doesn't inhibit detoxification enzyme CYP3A4) and telithromycin.

Therefore, to those who theorize that genetics, adrenals, lungs, foods (milk proteins, soy, and wheat), albumin, bilirubin, trypsin and alpha 1 antitrypsin provide contributing factors to the cause of autism, I say, "You Are Right!"

6 VACCINES THEORY

I intentionally discuss this theory last. This report lists so many possible contributing factors of autism that I hope I won't be accused of pointing the finger solely at vaccines.

Some vaccine theorists propose that vaccines may not be the primary cause of autism; rather, they conclude that vaccines might be the last straw or tipping point of the immune system. The medical community as a whole agrees that when an immunocompromised person is given a live virus vaccine, it could activate in them. Therefore, they sometimes recommend that immunocompromised people should not take live virus vaccines.

Do we think that autistic children are __not__ immunocompromised, therefore, this basic precaution does not apply?

What about all the upper respiratory infections, ear infections, GI issues, etc. for which these children need frequent treatments with antibiotics?

At what point is this considered immunocompromised?

This report theorizes that surfactants, albumin and hyperbilirubinemia may play roles in causing autism. I noticed that both surfactants and albumins are added to some vaccines as pharmacological adjuvants. Pharmacological adjuvants are used to enhance the body's immune response to an antigen. This, of course, could be just a coincidence, but it also may be something that deserves a closer look along with other adjuvants like aluminum added to vaccines.

Medical studies have proven that mercury has toxic effects on the human body. Aluminum, however, is under the radar, and there is not much awareness by the general public about its effect on the body. Aluminum is a neurotoxin that is known to down regulate the enzyme Glucose 6 phosphate dehydrogenase (G6Pd). As you remember G6Pdd is one of the hemolytic anemia disorders I discussed in chapter 5. My autistic son is G6Pd deficient (G6Pdd). G6Pdd is listed as a genetic condition that causes hemolysis or breakdown of red blood cells which can lead to internal bleeding and Kernicterus.

What might be the effects of injecting aluminum into a person with a genetically weak G6PD enzyme?

Would it down regulate this enzyme even more?
Would this down regulation increase risk of hemolysis?

G6Pdd or Glucose 6 phosphate dehydrogenase deficiency is listed as the most common enzyme deficiency in the world; however, most people who have it are never tested for it or diagnosed. My son was not diagnosed until he was 5 years old because he did not exhibit the classic symptoms. When thinking of G6Pdd most doctors look for children who look jaundiced and have severe hemolysis. My son was jaundiced as a baby, but did not exhibit any other noticeable symptoms as a child. He was diagnosed due to my research lead me in that direction when I theorized that my son's metabolic problems were partially centered in the Pentose Phosphate Pathway. I had read the work of Dr. Amy Yasko and thought the concept of metabolic roadblocks in relation to autism was an interesting theory. After studying the various enzymes in the Pentose Phosphate Pathway, I read that the G6Pd enzyme was the most common enzyme defect in the world, so I thought,

Why not start there?

I proposed the possibility of my son having G6Pdd to one of his doctors and was quickly informed there was no way he could have it. A year passed and my puzzle solving was stuck because this G6Pdd piece seemed lost. I decided to find a private lab that would test my son with their own doctor. The test results showed that he was indeed G6Pd deficient. I then took these lab results to my son's pediatrician who referred him to a hematologist at our local children's hospital. Because my son's G6Pd level was so low and he was asymptomatic the hematologist repeated the blood work just to make sure it wasn't a mistake. The results confirmed that my son was G6Pd deficient and he was officially diagnosed with Glucose 6 phosphate dehydrogenase deficiency.

This enzyme is important because it maintains the level of nicotinamide adenine dinucleotide phosphate (NADPH), which in turn maintains the level of glutathione in the body. Like many children with autism, my son's glutathione level is extremely low. Everyone needs glutathione in order to detoxify from toxins and chemicals, and it is extremely important to children's little bodies.

Therefore, wouldn't a G6PD deficient child exposed to high levels of surfactants/chemicals have an even more difficult time metabolizing them out?

This enzyme is also very important because a deficiency increases one's risk of red blood cell hemolysis (internal bleeding).

Knowing children's G6Pd enzyme functioning status could save lives by prevent unnecessary negative drug reactions. The quantitative test that checks the G6Pd enzyme level of function is usually less than $100. A long list of medications and substances contraindicated for a person who is G6Pd deficient includes sulfur containing drugs, certain antibiotics, blue dyes, fava beans, large doses of vitamin C, synthetic vitamin K (my son also received this within hours of birth), acetaminophen (fever reducer) and more. For a complete list of contraindicated medications and foods to avoid you may visit www.G6PDdeficiency.org and look under "living with G6Pd deficiency".

In the United States only certain states screen for G6Pdd during the newborn screening test. However even when screened the results aren't received until after they've already been given synthetic vitamin K. The state I live in does not screen for G6Pdd at birth, therefore my son was given so many drugs that he was never supposed to receive. From sulfur based antibiotics to synthetic vitamin K (given within hours of birth), to repeated courses of acetaminophen.

This makes me so sad, especially since I know it is happening to so many other children every day. Every state should add G6Pd screening to their newborn screening test.

Since natural Vitamin K is not the problem for infants with G6Pdd, only synthetic vitamin K, why can't these infants receive natural vitamin K instead? (No soy based products please since some infants could be sensitive).

Vitamin K is given at birth to prevent bleeding in the brain from hemorrhagic disorders like seen in Vitamin K deficiency. Synthetic Vitamin is given with hours of birth and has proven through statistics to save the lives of babies with hemorrhagic disease from bleeding to death. It is very ironic that synthetic Vitamin K would do the complete opposite to babies with G6Pdd a hemolytic anemic disorder that causes bleeding. Synthetic Vitamin K can cause hemolysis or bleeding in these G6Pdd babies.

Shouldn't we find a way to provide both types of babies the Vitamin K they need in a form that both their bodies can tolerate? Wouldn't natural Vitamin K be the answer?

One factor that connects G6Pdd and autism symptoms is jaundice. G6Pdd causes jaundice when red blood cell hemolysis occurs. A study in Denmark reported that babies who had jaundice were 67% more likely to develop autism.

Could pathological jaundice (caused by a disease or drug side effect) have been confused with physiological jaundice (normal part of development) in our children?

Was jaundice soon after birth their first cry for help, but no one heard them?

Surfactants and Vaccines – Synthetic and natural surfactants are used as adjuvants and/or as stabilizers of emulsions in vaccines.

What is the upper limit safe dosage of surfactant that can be added to vaccines without causing decreased cerebral perfusion and opening of the blood brain barrier?

What would happen if the surfactant dosage were raised to 100+ times the upper limit and added to a live virus vaccine or any vaccine?

Would this create an exaggerated response to that vaccine especially if the person had a genetic issue with surfactants?

Could this be what is happening with our excessive surfactant exposure?

Remember that some of these children were premature and received steroids at birth to increase surfactant production. Once born, they were exposed to surfactants every time they were bathed with soaps and had their diapers changed (baby wipes). They were also exposed every time we washed one of their cute little outfits in laundry detergent. Let's not forget tummy time, the accumulated exposure from crawling and walking on stain repellent carpet. Then there is the nursery, that beautifully theme-painted room with the cozy foam insulation in the walls. We can't leave out the surfactant laced fuel exhaust that our children are exposed to every time we take them for a walk, drive, or park in our attached garages. In addition, there are always those biosurfactant-producing bacteria from the frequent bacterial infections that lead to repeated antibiotic courses that welcome surfactant-creating Candidas fungal infections. This doesn't even include the surfactant exposure of the mother and how much she could have passed to her fetus in the womb.

Story after story from parents report that within days to weeks of receiving the last course of vaccines their children began to show signs that something was wrong. *Did something happen to the immune system?*

Was the act of giving vaccines to an immunocompromised child with an undiagnosed disorder which leads to hyperbilirubinemia, plus exposure to high levels of environmental surfactants and antibiotics the straw that broke the camel's (immune system) back?

Since vaccines have ingredients that include egg protein (albumen and albumin), soy protein (albumin), cow albumin, and human albumin, could albumin allergy also be an issue?

Could this allergy have reduced how bilirubin was bound and removed from the body? Could this reaction have also created autoimmune hemolytic anemia leading to bilirubin encephalopathy?

Consider, also, the acetaminophen autism theory. It proposes that giving acetaminophen directly after vaccines lowers glutathione levels making it more difficult for the body to detoxify the vaccine components.

How low might glutathione levels go if an already G6Pd deficient child receives a vaccine with aluminum in it, and is also given acetaminophen?

I was instructed to give my son acetaminophen as fever prevention for the first 24 hours after receiving his vaccines. (He hadn't yet been diagnosed with G6Pd deficiency.)

This situation is a mess—physically, emotionally, socially, politically, and financially. People are afraid to say anything negative about vaccines because they might be accused of causing an epidemic.

The irony is that those who decline vaccines for their children are seeking answers regarding the current autism epidemic. Though ignored, vaccine injury is real. Whether vaccine injury can be applied to the autism epidemic is still to be determined. The general public should know that most parents who decline vaccinations do so, not because they are against vaccines, but because the scientific community has not found definitive and preventable contributing causes of autism. These parents are choosing to side with caution until the truth is found.

Whether-or-not-to-vaccinate is too serious a subject to flippantly say, "You Are Right!" However, in light of the new surfactant, albumin, bilirubin and aluminum connections uncovered in this report, if you theorize that vaccines are a contributing cause of autism, "You Are Right" to keep them on your suspect list.

More research definitely must be done.

R M Terry

7 WHAT THIS ALL MEANS

Like the habitat of Zombie Alligators, our global habitat has obviously been compromised. Rates of autism vary from state to state, province to province and country to country. One region may have extremely high rates of autism and the region next to it may have low rates of autism.

Why?

Globally Asia Pacific dominates the surfactant manufacturing market, followed by North America, then Europe. My hope is that a survey will be done which compares gross surfactant production by state, province and country with the incidence of autism in those areas to see if there is a correlation. I also hope this survey will assess the different types of surfactants produced in case there is a greater incidence of autism with a certain type of surfactant instead of all surfactants (anionic, cationic, amphoteric, and nonionic). I also hope that hemolytic blood disorders, liver disorders causing hyperbilirubinemia, disorders that cause hypoalbuminemia and drugs routinely given to infants that bind albumin will be analyzed.

One of the biggest concerns that society should have regarding our excessive level of surfactant exposure is that surfactants help chemicals to absorb. This concern remains whether a company uses a brand that degrades in one month or in five years. The damage to our health is immediate upon exposure. Considering our high chemical exposure levels,

Is there any wonder there is an Autism Epidemic, an Allergy Epidemic, an Asthma Epidemic, a Cancer Epidemic, and an Autoimmune Epidemic, or an increase in disorders like Lupus, Fibromyalgia, Multiple Sclerosis, Arthritis, and Chronic Bronchitis?

This book was written, not because I know how to cure autism, not because I've figured it all out—only that I have found some common factors in the most common autism theories that have completed my autism puzzle. My hope is that this research warrants another look by all who are trying to solve their autism puzzle. You are right, I am right, and they are right. In the big scheme of things it doesn't really matter who is right because our children are still autistic. Perhaps when everyone becomes open to others' theories, we can brainstorm a solution to help these children. You know the saying, "It takes a village to raise a child": it is going to take a village of open-minded parents, doctors, and scientists who are willing to re-analyze the data and stop definitively ruling out possible causes just because the alternative would be too expensive or politically incorrect.

If a subset of the population is sensitive to <u>any</u> of the components in vaccines, don't they deserve a screening tool that protects them <u>before</u> vaccines are given?

I'm personally not asking or expecting anyone to get rid of vaccines; I however don't think a screening tool is too much to ask.

My personal position on vaccines is I'm definitely pro-vaccines for those people that aren't sensitive to them. I am grateful to everyone that feels strongly about the need for vaccines because herd immunity is what is keeping the rest of us safe.

So if there was a demonstration march regarding vaccines, you'd see me carrying two signs. One for the people that say we have to take them to keep epidemics at bay and another that says people who may be sensitive deserve to have a screening test that protects them.

My personal stance on all pharmaceutical drugs is the less is more approach.
Therefore I think it is important to add that even though I am pro vaccines for those people who aren't sensitive to them I do believe that the <u>amount</u> of vaccines given before a child is 5 years old has gotten out of hand.

More work must be done.

You can see how surfactants affect our lungs, immune system, chemical exposure, cerebral perfusion, blood brain barrier, muscle tone, fatty acids, phospholipids, and more. My hope is that this surfactant/albumin/bilirubin connection will catapult theories into real medical diagnoses for our children.

To the many doctors and scientists who are ready and able to take this information and create viable tests and treatment plans for children with autism, I look forward to seeing what you can do and saying *"You Are Right"*!

Share your thoughts at www.YouWereRight.org or email me at Autism@YouWereRight.org .

ABOUT THE AUTHOR

R.M. Terry is the mother of an 8-year-old son who has been diagnosed with autism. She has dedicated the last six years to research autism in order to help her son and other children with autism. She has always had an interest in and passion for science and medicine. Her life's goal is simple: do whatever she can to help children with autism and their families by increasing awareness regarding this disorder.

You can stay updated on what she is doing and join the conversation by visiting www.YouWereRight.org .

A book club expands personal literary experiences by providing a platform for an open exchange of opinions. As an author trying to increase public awareness of autism, I can't think of a better forum for exposing this devastating disorder and its possible causes. RM Terry

Book club discussion questions for

Autism Theories Dissected, You Are Right!

1. What is this book about? What motivated the author to write this book?

2. What did you know about autism before reading this book? Has reading this book changed how you view autism? Do you know any families affected by autism?

3. What autism theories had you heard of before reading this book? Did you agree with any of these theories? Why? Do you think the author connected the common autism theories? Do you feel like you learned anything useful? Was the medical information hard to follow?

4. What is a surfactant? Had you ever heard the word *surfactant* before reading this book? What products do you use every day have surfactants in them? Does your family's level of surfactant exposure concern you? If you did the survey assessing how many surfactant filled products are in your home, how many did you find?

5. Were you surprised to learn that vaccines contain adjuvants such as surfactants, albumin, and aluminum? Should there be a screening tool to protect people sensitive to the ingredients in vaccines? Should the general public be concerned or is this just anti-vaccine propaganda?

6. Do you know any brand of laundry detergent, bath soap, or shampoo that is surfactant-free?

7. Does the saying "if it looks like a duck and quacks like a duck it's probably a duck" apply to the bilirubin encephalopathy theory since bilirubin encephalopathy looks exactly like autism?

8. What is Glucose 6 phosphate dehydrogenase deficiency (G6PDD)? Why would having it be a problem for a person exposed to toxins and chemicals?

9. Do you read product labels before you buy? Do you have any concerns when you see long chemical names that you don't recognize? Why?

10. What did you like/dislike about this book? How did this book affect you? What outcome do you hope results because of this book?

If you are a book club moderator and would like to ask questions before or after your discussion of this book, you may contact me at bookclub@YouWereRight.org or visit www.YouWereRight.org. I welcome your questions.

Let's start the discussion!

www.ingramcontent.com/pod-product-compliance
Lightning Source LLC
Chambersburg PA
CBHW071330310526
45789CB00017B/2177